Sharon Cooper - Jones

Broken to Beautiful:

Healing Emotional Baggage for Single Women

FROM BROKEN TO BEAUTIFUL : HEALING EMOTIONAL BAGGAGE FOR SINGLE WOMEN

First edition. February 11, 2024.

Copyright © 2024 Sharon Cooper-Jones.

ISBN: 979-8224274277

Written by Sharon Cooper-Jones.

Table of Contents

From Broken to Beautiful: Healing Emotional Baggage for Single Women

Chapter 1: Understanding Emotional Baggage

Denying Emotional Baggage

In the journey of healing emotional baggage, it is essential to understand what emotional baggage truly means. It refers to the unresolved emotions, traumas, and negative experiences that we carry from our past, often hindering personal growth and hindering us from living our lives to the fullest. Single women, like many others, may find themselves burdened by this emotional baggage, affecting their relationships, self-esteem, and overall happiness.

Healing from past trauma is an integral part of this process. Unresolved traumas can stem from various experiences, such as abuse, neglect, or any other form of emotional or physical harm. These traumas can leave deep scars that influence our behavior, choices, and relationships. Acknowledging and accepting these traumas is the first step towards healing and overcoming their effects on our lives.

Childhood issues can also play a significant role in emotional baggage. Our upbringing shapes our beliefs, values, and patterns of behavior. Negative experiences during childhood, such as a lack of love or emotional support, can lead to feelings of unworthiness and insecurities in adulthood. Understanding and coping with these childhood wounds allows us to break free from the patterns that may be holding us back.

Heartbreak and failed relationships are often significant contributors to emotional baggage. The pain and disappointment of past relationships can create a fear of vulnerability and intimacy. Overcoming these heartbreaks requires learning to trust again, setting healthy boundaries, and realizing that each relationship failure is an opportunity for growth and self-discovery.

Grief and loss are emotions that we all experience at some point in our lives. Whether it's the loss of a loved one, a job, or a dream, these losses can leave profound emotional scars. Navigating through grief involves giving ourselves permission to mourn, seeking support, and finding healthy ways to honor our losses while gradually embracing the present and the future.

Phobias and fears can act as roadblocks to personal growth and fulfillment. These can be rooted in past experiences or childhood traumas and can manifest in various ways, such as fear of commitment, fear of abandonment, or social anxiety. Confronting and overcoming these phobias and fears is a crucial step towards emotional freedom and creating a more fulfilling life.

Understanding and defining emotional baggage is the first step towards healing. It involves acknowledging the impact of past traumas, childhood issues, failed relationships, grief, and phobias on our lives. By addressing these areas, single women can embark on a journey of healing, self-discovery, and personal growth. In the upcoming chapters, we will provide practical strategies and tools to help you navigate through these challenges, break free from emotional baggage, and transform your life from broken to beautiful.

Identifying the Types of Emotional Baggage

In our journey towards healing and personal growth, it is crucial for single women to identify and understand the types of emotional baggage they may be carrying. Emotional baggage can be defined as unresolved emotions, trauma, or negative experiences from the past that continue to affect our present lives and relationships. By recognizing and acknowledging these issues, we can begin the process of healing and transforming our lives from broken to beautiful.

1. Healing from past trauma: Many single women may have experienced various forms of trauma in their lives, such as physical or emotional abuse, neglect, or traumatic events. It is essential to recognize how these experiences have shaped our beliefs, behaviors, and relationships. By seeking professional help or joining support groups, we can begin to heal and release the emotional burden we carry.

2. Coping with childhood issues: Our childhood experiences often shape our adult lives, and unresolved childhood issues can manifest as emotional baggage. Single women may have grown up in dysfunctional families, experienced parental divorce, or faced other challenges that impact their self esteem and relationships. By addressing these issues through therapy or self reflection, we can develop healthier coping mechanisms and break negative patterns.

From Broken to Beautiful: Healing Emotional Baggage for Single Women

From Broken to Beautiful: Healing Emotional Baggage for Single Women

3. Overcoming heartbreak and failed relationships: Heartbreak and failed relationships can leave deep emotional scars. It is important for single women to recognize any lingering pain, resentment, or fear that may arise from these experiences. By forgiving ourselves and others, learning from past mistakes, and focusing on self-love and growth, we can let go of emotional baggage and open ourselves to new possibilities.

4. Dealing with grief and loss: Loss is an inevitable part of life, and the grieving process can be challenging for single women. Whether it is the loss of a loved one, a job, or a dream, it is essential to honor our emotions and allow ourselves to heal. Seeking support from loved ones, therapy, or grief support groups can provide a safe space to navigate through the grieving process and release emotional baggage.

5. Navigating through phobias and fears: Phobias and fears can hold us back from living fulfilling lives. Single women may have developed phobias or fears due to past traumatic experiences or negative beliefs. By identifying these fears and seeking professional help, we can work towards overcoming them and reclaiming our power.

Recognizing and understanding the types of emotional baggage we carry is the first step towards healing and transformation. By addressing these issues, single women can break free from the limitations of their past and create a future filled with love, joy, and fulfillment. Remember, you are not defined by your emotional baggage, but rather by your strength and resilience in overcoming it.

Recognizing the Impact of Emotional Baggage on Single Women

Emotional baggage can weigh heavily on the hearts and minds of single women, hindering their ability to find happiness and fulfillment in both personal and romantic relationships. Whether stemming from past trauma, childhood issues, heartbreak, grief, phobias, or fears, these emotional burdens can have a profound impact on every aspect of a woman's life.

Understanding the effects of emotional baggage is the first step towards healing and reclaiming one's life. It is crucial for single women to recognize that their past experiences shape their present reality, and that healing is possible. This subchapter aims to shed light on the various ways emotional baggage can manifest and provide insights into how to navigate these challenges.

One of the key areas this subchapter explores is healing from past trauma. Many single women carry deep scars from past experiences, such as abuse, neglect, or betrayal. These wounds can affect their self-esteem, trust in others, and ability to form healthy relationships. By acknowledging these traumas and seeking professional help or support groups, women can begin to untangle the emotional knots that are holding them back.

Coping with childhood issues is another crucial aspect that single women must address. Childhood experiences, such as dysfunctional family dynamics or neglect, can create emotional baggage that impacts their adult lives. Recognizing these patterns and seeking therapy can help single women break free from negative cycles and establish healthier ways of relating to themselves and others.

Heartbreak and failed relationships can also leave deep emotional scars. It is essential for single women to acknowledge their pain and allow themselves to grieve. By doing so, they can begin to heal and move forward, opening themselves up to the possibility of healthier and more fulfilling relationships in the future.

Dealing with grief and loss is another important topic within this subchapter. Single women may face different types of loss, such as the death of a loved one or the end of a significant relationship. Learning healthy coping mechanisms and finding support from friends, family, or grief counseling can help women navigate through these difficult times.

Lastly, the subchapter explores the significance of addressing phobias and fears. Many single women carry around irrational fears that hold them back from pursuing their dreams or engaging in fulfilling relationships. By identifying and confronting these fears, women can break free from self imposed limitations and embrace a life of courage and empowerment.

In conclusion, emotional baggage can have a significant impact on the lives of single women, affecting their ability to find happiness and fulfillment. Recognizing the various ways emotional baggage manifests and seeking appropriate support is crucial for healing. By addressing past trauma, childhood issues, heartbreak, grief, and fears, single women can begin their journey from broken to beautiful, reclaiming their lives and opening themselves up to a future filled with love, joy, and emotional well-being.

Chapter 2: Healing from Past Trauma

Exploring the Role of Past Trauma in Emotional Baggage

In our journey from brokenness to beauty, it is essential for single women to understand the profound impact that past trauma can have on our emotional baggage. Often, the experiences we have endured in our childhood or past relationships leave lasting imprints on our hearts and minds, shaping the way we view ourselves, others, and the world around us.

Healing from past trauma is a crucial step towards freeing ourselves from the weight of emotional baggage that can hinder our personal growth and happiness. It is important to recognize that trauma comes in many forms, whether it be physical, emotional, or psychological. Childhood abuse, neglect, or witnessing traumatic events can leave deep wounds that affect our relationships, self-esteem, and overall emotional well-being.

Coping with childhood issues is a complex process that requires patience, self compassion, and professional guidance. By acknowledging and working through these issues, we can begin to understand their impact on our present lives and develop healthier coping mechanisms. It is through this healing journey that we can break free from the chains of the past and pave the way for a brighter future.

Heartbreak and failed relationships can also contribute to our emotional baggage. When we invest our love and trust in someone, only to have that trust shattered, it can leave lasting scars. It is crucial to recognize that healing from these wounds takes time and self-reflection. By understanding our patterns and beliefs that may have contributed to these failed relationships, we can grow and learn from our experiences, ultimately attracting healthier and more fulfilling connections.

Grief and loss are universal experiences that touch all of our lives at some point. Whether it is the loss of a loved one, a dream, or a significant life change, navigating through these emotions can be incredibly challenging. By allowing ourselves to grieve and seeking support from others, we can begin to heal and find solace in the memories and lessons our losses have taught us.

Lastly, phobias and fears can create barriers in our lives, preventing us from fully embracing new experiences and opportunities. Identifying the root causes of these fears and seeking professional help can empower us to overcome them. Through gradual exposure and implementing healthy coping strategies, we can reclaim our lives and step into a future filled with courage and resilience.

Understanding the role of past trauma in our emotional baggage is a vital step in our journey towards healing and transformation. By addressing these issues head-on, single women can embark on a path of self-discovery, growth, and ultimately, finding the beauty that lies within. Remember, you are not alone on this journey, and there is hope for a brighter future beyond your past.

Understanding the Healing Process

Healing is a journey that each of us must embark on at some point in our lives. For single women, healing becomes even more crucial as we navigate the complexities of emotional baggage, past trauma, childhood issues, heartbreak, failed relationships, grief, loss, phobias, and fears. In this subchapter, we will explore the various aspects of the healing process and provide guidance and support to help you transform from broken to beautiful.

Healing emotional baggage is the first step towards achieving inner peace and happiness. It involves acknowledging and addressing the wounds that have accumulated over time, often as a result of past experiences. By understanding the root causes of our emotional baggage, we can begin to release its hold on us and create space for healing and growth.

When it comes to healing from past trauma, it is essential to approach the process with compassion and patience. Traumatic experiences can leave deep scars that may take time to heal. By seeking professional help, engaging in self care practices, and surrounding ourselves with a supportive community, we can gradually overcome the impact of trauma and reclaim our lives.

Coping with childhood issues requires a deep dive into our upbringing and the patterns that have shaped our adult lives. Through therapy, journaling, and self reflection, we can gain insights into the wounds inflicted during our formative years and develop strategies to heal them.

Heartbreak and failed relationships can leave us feeling shattered and vulnerable. However, by understanding our worth and setting healthy boundaries, we can learn valuable lessons from these experiences. Healing from heartbreak involves self-love, forgiveness, and a commitment to personal growth.

Grief and loss are natural parts of life, but they can be overwhelming. By allowing ourselves to grieve, seeking support, and engaging in healing practices such as meditation and creative expression, we can navigate through the pain and find solace.

Phobias and fears can hold us back from living our lives to the fullest. By gradually exposing ourselves to our fears, seeking professional help, and practicing self-compassion, we can conquer these limiting beliefs and embrace a life of courage and freedom.

Understanding the healing process is not a linear journey but rather a cyclical one. It requires self-reflection, self-compassion, and a commitment to personal growth. As single women, we have the power to transform our pain into strength, our wounds into wisdom, and our brokenness into beauty. By embarking on this healing journey, we can reclaim our lives and create a brighter future filled with love, joy, and fulfillment.

Seeking Professional Help and Support

In the journey from brokenness to beauty, seeking professional help and support is a vital step for single women dealing with emotional baggage, healing from past trauma, coping with childhood issues, overcoming heartbreak and failed relationships, dealing with grief and loss, and navigating through phobias and fears. This subchapter aims to shed light on the importance of seeking professional guidance and the various avenues available for support.

Emotional baggage can weigh heavily on a person's mental and emotional well-being. It is crucial for single women to recognize when their emotional wounds are too deep to heal on their own. Seeking the assistance of a professional therapist or counselor can provide a safe space to explore these emotional challenges, process past experiences, and develop effective coping mechanisms.

Healing from past trauma requires a delicate approach, as the scars left behind can be profound. Working with a trauma-informed therapist can enable single women to navigate through their traumatic experiences, gradually heal, and reclaim their power. These trained professionals can guide individuals through evidence-based therapies such as cognitive-behavioral therapy (CBT) or eye movement desensitization and reprocessing (EMDR), helping them regain control over their lives.

Coping with childhood issues is often a complex and sensitive process. Seeking professional help, such as working with a licensed child psychologist or counselor, can assist single women in unraveling the impact of their past and understanding how it affects their present. These professionals employ a variety of therapeutic techniques tailored to address childhood wounds, allowing individuals to break free from negative patterns and create healthier relationships.

Overcoming heartbreak and failed relationships can leave deep emotional scars. Engaging with a relationship coach or therapist who specializes in this area can provide valuable guidance and support. These professionals can help single women navigate their emotions, rebuild self-esteem, and develop healthier relationship patterns.

Dealing with grief and loss is an inevitable part of life, and seeking professional help is essential during this challenging time. Grief counselors or therapists can provide a compassionate, non-judgmental space for single women to process their emotions, find meaning in their loss, and gradually rebuild their lives.

Navigating through phobias and fears can be overwhelming and limit personal growth. Seeking the assistance of a trained professional, such as a licensed psychologist or therapist specializing in anxiety disorders, can empower single women to overcome their fears. Through various therapeutic techniques, these professionals can help individuals challenge their irrational beliefs, develop coping strategies, and ultimately reclaim their lives from the grip of fear.

In conclusion, seeking professional help and support is a crucial step for single women on the path from brokenness to beauty. Whether dealing with emotional baggage, past trauma, childhood issues, heartbreak, grief, or phobias, professional guidance can provide the tools and support necessary for healing and growth. Remember, you don't have to face these challenges alone – reaching out for help is a sign of strength and self-care.

Chapter 3: Coping with Childhood Issues

Uncovering Childhood Emotional Baggage

Childhood is often seen as a time of innocence, joy, and carefree moments. However, for many single women, it can also be a time of emotional baggage that can hinder personal growth and hinder the ability to form healthy relationships. In this subchapter, we will delve into the depths of childhood emotional baggage and explore ways to heal from past trauma, cope with childhood issues, and overcome heartbreak and failed relationships.

Childhood experiences shape who we are as adults, and unfortunately, not all of these experiences are positive. Emotional trauma, neglect, abuse, or even witnessing dysfunctional relationships can leave lasting scars on our hearts and minds. This baggage can manifest in various ways, such as fear of intimacy, low self-esteem, trust issues, or difficulty forming healthy attachments.

Healing from past trauma is a journey that requires self-reflection, self compassion, and professional help if needed. It involves acknowledging and accepting the pain, understanding its impact on our lives, and actively working towards letting go of the negative emotions associated with it. Through therapy, support groups, or self-help techniques, single women can learn to reframe their past experiences and develop healthier coping mechanisms.

Childhood issues can also resurface in adult relationships, causing patterns of heartbreak and failed relationships. Unresolved conflicts or unmet needs from childhood can lead to self-sabotaging behaviors or attracting partners who mirror the negative dynamics experienced in the past. By recognizing these patterns and seeking therapy or counseling, single women can break free from these cycles and create healthier relationship dynamics.

Dealing with grief and loss is another aspect of childhood emotional baggage that single women may face. Loss of a parent, sibling, or caregiver can have a profound impact on emotional well-being and may require professional help to navigate through the grieving process.

Navigating through phobias and fears that stem from childhood experiences can be challenging but not impossible. With the help of therapy and gradual exposure, single women can confront their fears, understand their origins, and develop strategies to overcome them.

Uncovering childhood emotional baggage is a crucial step towards healing and creating a brighter future. By acknowledging the impact of past experiences, single women can empower themselves to break free from negative patterns and build healthier, more fulfilling lives. Remember, you are not defined by your past, but rather by your ability to heal and grow from it.

Healing Inner Child Wounds

In our journey towards emotional healing, it is essential to address the wounds of our inner child. As single women, we may have experienced various forms of emotional baggage that stem from our past traumas and childhood issues. These wounds can manifest themselves in our relationships, heartbreaks, and even our ability to cope with grief and loss. However, by acknowledging and healing our inner child wounds, we can break free from the cycle of emotional pain and create a beautiful future for ourselves.

Childhood experiences play a significant role in shaping our beliefs, behaviors, and patterns in adulthood. Negative experiences, such as abandonment, neglect, abuse, or witnessing conflict, can leave deep scars on our inner child. These wounds may manifest as fear, low self-esteem, trust issues, or difficulties in forming healthy relationships. To heal these wounds, we must first understand and accept the impact they have had on us.

Healing our inner child wounds requires compassion, patience, and self reflection. It involves revisiting the past, acknowledging the pain, love and understanding to our younger selves. By nurturing our inner child, we can create a safe space within us where healing can take place. This process allows us to release the negative emotions associated with past traumas and transform our perspective on ourselves and our relationships.

Coping with childhood issues is a crucial step in our emotional healing journey. It involves identifying patterns that no longer serve us and replacing them with healthier coping mechanisms. Seeking therapy or support groups can provide a safe environment to explore these issues and gain valuable insights from others who have experienced similar struggles.

Overcoming heartbreak and failed relationships is another area where healing our inner child wounds is vital. By understanding how our past experiences may have influenced our choices in partners or our ability to trust, we can break free from unhealthy patterns. This process allows us to create healthier boundaries, develop self-love, and attract healthier relationships in the future.

Dealing with grief and loss can be particularly challenging for single women, as we may feel the weight of our emotions alone. Healing our inner child wounds in this area involves giving ourselves permission to grieve, seeking support from loved ones or grief counseling, and finding healthy ways to honor our losses. By allowing ourselves to feel and heal, we can navigate through grief and loss with greater resilience and strength.

Navigating through phobias and fears is yet another aspect of healing our inner child wounds. Childhood experiences can create deep-rooted fears that hold us back from fully embracing life. By confronting and challenging these fears, we can regain our power and live more authentically. Therapy, mindfulness practices, and gradual exposure techniques can be effective tools in overcoming phobias and fears.

Healing our inner child wounds is a transformative process that requires dedication and self-compassion. By acknowledging and addressing our emotional baggage, we can break free from the cycle of pain and create a beautiful future for ourselves. Through healing, we can empower ourselves as single women, embrace our worth, and attract the love and happiness we deserve.

Releasing Limiting Beliefs and Patterns

In our journey from brokenness to beauty, one of the key steps we must take is to release the limiting beliefs and patterns that hold us back. As single women, we often carry emotional baggage from past experiences, trauma, childhood issues, heartbreak, failed relationships, grief, loss, phobias, and fears. These burdens can weigh us down, prevent us from moving forward, and hinder our ability to find true happiness and fulfillment.

To begin the process of healing, we must first acknowledge and identify the limiting beliefs and patterns that have become ingrained within us. These beliefs can manifest as negative self-talk, self-doubt, fear of intimacy, fear of abandonment, fear of failure, or a general feeling of unworthiness. By shining a light on these beliefs, we can begin to understand how they have shaped our lives and recognize the impact they have on our ability to find love and happiness.

Once we have identified these limiting beliefs, we can begin the process of releasing them. This can be done through various therapeutic techniques such as cognitive-behavioral therapy, mindfulness practices, journaling, or working with a trusted therapist or coach. It is important to remember that healing is a personal journey, and what works for one person may not work for another. Finding the right approach for you is essential.

Releasing these beliefs and patterns requires courage and self-compassion. It may involve facing painful memories, confronting fears, and challenging long held beliefs about ourselves and relationships. However, by doing so, we can begin to break free from the chains that have held us back and open ourselves up to new possibilities.

As we release these limiting beliefs and patterns, we create space for healing and growth. We can cultivate a new sense of self-worth, self-love, and self acceptance. We can learn to trust ourselves and others again, and to believe that we are deserving of love and happiness.

In this subchapter, we will explore various techniques and strategies for releasing limiting beliefs and patterns. We will delve into the healing process, providing practical exercises and guidance for single women who are ready to let go of their emotional baggage and transform their lives. Together, we will embark on a journey of self-discovery, empowerment, and transformation, as we move from brokenness to beautiful.

Chapter 4: Overcoming Heartbreak and Failed Relationships Processing the Pain of Heartbreak

Heartbreak is a universal experience that can leave us feeling shattered, lost, and utterly broken. Whether it's the end of a long-term relationship, a failed marriage, or the loss of a loved one, the pain can be overwhelming. In this subchapter, we will explore the various ways in which single women can process the pain of heartbreak and begin their journey towards healing and self-discovery.

The first step in processing heartbreak is acknowledging and accepting the pain. It's crucial to allow yourself to feel the emotions that arise, whether it's anger, sadness, or confusion. Give yourself permission to grieve the loss and understand that it is a necessary part of healing.

Once you have acknowledged your pain, it's essential to create a support system. Surround yourself with friends, family, or a therapist who can provide a safe space for you to express your emotions without judgment. Sharing your feelings with others can bring comfort and provide a fresh perspective on your situation.

Another vital aspect of processing heartbreak is self-care. Take time to focus on your physical, emotional, and mental well-being. Engage in activities that bring you joy and help you reconnect with yourself. This could include exercise, journaling, meditation, or pursuing hobbies that you love. By taking care of yourself, you are allowing yourself to heal and rebuild.

Additionally, it's crucial to react to the lessons learned from the experience. Heartbreak can over valuable insights into ourselves and our patterns in relationships. Take the opportunity to evaluate what went wrong and identify any patterns or behaviors that may have contributed to the outcome. This self reflection will help you grow and avoid making the same mistakes in the future.

Finally, it's important to have patience with yourself. Healing from heartbreak takes time, and everyone's journey is unique. Be gentle with yourself as you navigate through the waves of emotions and remember that healing is a process.

In conclusion, processing the pain of heartbreak is a challenging yet essential part of healing emotional baggage for single women. By acknowledging and accepting the pain, creating a support system, practicing self-care, reflecting on lessons learned, and having patience, you can begin your journey from broken to beautiful. Remember, you are resilient, and with time and self-love, you will emerge stronger and ready for a new chapter in your life.

Learning from Failed Relationships

In our journey through life, it is inevitable that we will encounter failed relationships. Whether it is a heartbreak from a romantic partner, a broken friendship, or a strained family dynamic, these experiences can leave us with emotional baggage that weighs us down. However, it is essential for single women to understand that these failed relationships can provide valuable lessons and opportunities for growth.

One of the first steps in healing emotional baggage is acknowledging the impact of past trauma and identifying its source. Failed relationships often trigger unresolved childhood issues and can unearth deep-seated fears and phobias. By recognizing these patterns, we can begin to understand the root causes of our emotional wounds and work towards healing them.

Coping with childhood issues is an integral part of healing from failed relationships. Understanding how our past experiences shape our present behaviors can empower us to break free from negative patterns. Through therapy, support groups, or self-reflection exercises, we can learn healthy coping mechanisms and develop a better understanding of ourselves.

Overcoming heartbreak and failed relationships requires time and self compassion. It is crucial to allow ourselves to grieve and process the loss. Only by acknowledging our pain can we begin to heal. This subchapter will provide strategies to navigate through the stages of grief and over tools to rebuild self esteem and self-worth.

Dealing with grief and loss is a universal experience, and it is important to remember that we are not alone in our struggles. Connecting with others who have experienced similar pain can provide a sense of comfort and support. This subchapter will explore the benefits of support groups, counseling, and seeking solace in friendships and community.

Navigating through phobias and fears can be challenging, but it is possible with the right tools. This subchapter will delve into various techniques, such as exposure therapy and cognitive-behavioral therapy, to help single women overcome their fears and regain control over their lives.

Learning from failed relationships is a transformative process that can lead to personal growth and self-discovery. By addressing our emotional baggage and healing from past trauma, we can break free from negative patterns and create

healthier relationships in the future. Through self-reflection, therapy, and support, single women can move from a place of brokenness to beauty, embracing their worth and finding fulfillment in their lives.

Building Healthy Relationship Patterns

In the journey of healing emotional baggage, single women often find themselves facing a myriad of challenges. From coping with past trauma and childhood issues to overcoming heartbreak and failed relationships, navigating through phobias and fears, and dealing with grief and loss, the path towards building healthy relationship patterns can seem daunting. However, it is crucial to remember that it is possible to transform from broken to beautiful, and create a fulfilling and loving partnership.

One of the first steps in building healthy relationship patterns is to recognize and heal from past trauma. Many single women carry emotional baggage that stems from painful experiences in their past. It is important to acknowledge these wounds and seek professional help if necessary. By addressing and processing these traumas, women can begin to let go of the negative patterns they may have developed as a result, and open themselves up to healthier and more balanced relationships.

Coping with childhood issues is another vital aspect of building healthy relationship patterns. Our formative years greatly influence our adult relationships, and unresolved childhood issues can sabotage our chances of finding and maintaining a healthy partnership. Exploring these issues through therapy, support groups, or self-reflection can bring about a deeper understanding of oneself and help to break destructive relationship patterns.

Overcoming heartbreak and failed relationships is an essential part of the healing journey. It is natural to feel hurt and betrayed after a breakup, but dwelling on past pain can prevent us from moving forward. By learning to let go, forgiving ourselves and others, and focusing on personal growth, single women can break free from the chains of heartbreak and create space for new, healthy relationships to flourish.

Dealing with grief and loss is an inevitable part of life, and it can greatly impact our ability to form and maintain healthy relationships. It is important to give yourself permission to grieve and seek support from loved ones or professional counselors during these difficult times. By allowing ourselves to heal from loss, we can create a solid foundation for future relationships and prevent our grief from overshadowing our ability to connect with others.

Navigating through phobias and fears is yet another challenge that can hinder the development of healthy relationship patterns. These fears, whether rooted in past experiences or irrational beliefs, can prevent us from opening ourselves up to love and vulnerability. By gradually facing these fears, seeking therapy, and practicing self-compassion, single women can overcome their phobias and create space for love and connection in their lives.

In conclusion, building healthy relationship patterns is a multifaceted process that requires self-reflection, healing from past traumas, coping with childhood issues, overcoming heartbreak and failed relationships, dealing with grief and

loss, as well as navigating through phobias and fears. By embarking on this journey of self-discovery and growth, single women can transform from broken to beautiful, and create the fulfilling and loving partnerships they deserve.

Chapter 5: Dealing with Grief and Loss

Understanding the Stages of Grief

Grief is a universal human experience that we all encounter at some point in our lives. Whether it's the loss of a loved one, the end of a relationship, or even the loss of a dream, grief can be incredibly painful and overwhelming. As single women, we may often find ourselves grappling with grief in various forms. In this subchapter, we will explore the stages of grief and how understanding them can help us navigate through this difficult journey.

The stages of grief, as identified by psychiatrist Elisabeth Kübler-Ross, are denial, anger, bargaining, depression, and acceptance. It's important to note that these stages are not linear and can overlap or occur in a different order for each individual. By understanding these stages, we can gain insight into our own grieving process and find ways to heal our emotional baggage.

Denial is often the first stage of grief, where we may find it hard to believe or accept that the loss has occurred. This stage can be characterized by shock, numbness, and a sense of disbelief. It's essential to give ourselves permission to acknowledge our feelings and gradually move towards acceptance.

Anger is a natural response to grief and can manifest in various ways. We may feel anger towards ourselves, others, or even towards the person or situation that caused the loss. It's crucial to express and process this anger in healthy ways, such as through journaling, talking to a trusted friend, or seeking professional help if needed.

Bargaining is the stage where we may find ourselves trying to make deals or negotiate with a higher power to undo the loss. We may question what we could have done differently or make promises in hopes of reversing the situation. It's important to recognize that bargaining is a normal part of the grieving process, but ultimately, acceptance is necessary for healing.

Depression is a stage where we may experience intense sadness, hopelessness, and a sense of emptiness. It's crucial to seek support during this stage, whether it's through therapy, support groups, or leaning on trusted friends and family. Taking care of ourselves physically, emotionally, and mentally is essential during this phase.

Finally, acceptance is the stage where we come to terms with the loss and begin to rebuild our lives. It doesn't mean that we forget or stop missing what we have lost, but rather that we find a way to integrate the loss into our new reality. Acceptance allows us to move forward with hope and resilience.

Understanding the stages of grief can be a valuable tool in our journey of healing emotional baggage. By recognizing and honoring our feelings, seeking support, and giving ourselves time and space to grieve, we can gradually move towards acceptance and find beauty in our brokenness. Remember, healing takes time, and it's okay to seek help along the way. You are not alone in this journey.

Navigating the Loss of a Loved One

Losing a loved one is undoubtedly one of the most challenging and painful experiences we can face in life. The grief and heartache that accompany such a loss can be overwhelming, leaving us feeling lost and unsure of how to move forward. In this subchapter, we will explore the various emotions and challenges that arise when we are confronted with the loss of a loved one, and discuss strategies for navigating through this difficult time.

Grief is a complex and personal journey, and it is important to acknowledge and honor our own unique process. It is normal to experience a range of emotions, from sadness and anger to guilt and confusion. Understanding that these emotions are a natural part of the grieving process can help us to navigate through them with more compassion and self-acceptance.

One of the key aspects of healing from the loss of a loved one is allowing ourselves to grieve. It is essential to give ourselves permission to feel and express our emotions in a safe and supportive environment. This might involve seeking the support of a therapist, joining a grief support group, or conditioning on a trusted friend or family member. By sharing our pain and memories with others, we can find solace and strength in community.

Coping with the loss of a loved one also requires self-care. During times of grief, it is crucial to prioritize our physical, emotional, and spiritual well-being. Engaging in activities that bring us joy and comfort, such as exercise, meditation, or engaging in creative pursuits, can help to alleviate some of the pain and provide a sense of relief.

Additionally, it is important to acknowledge that healing takes time and that there is no right or wrong way to grieve. Each individual navigates the loss of a loved one dierently, and what works for one person may not work for another. It is essential to be patient and compassionate with ourselves as we navigate through this difficult journey.

In conclusion, the loss of a loved one is a painful and challenging experience. However, by acknowledging and honoring our emotions, seeking support, practicing self-care, and being patient with ourselves, we can navigate through the grief and eventually find healing. Remember, you are not alone in your journey, and there is hope for a brighter tomorrow.

Finding Meaning and Moving Forward

In the journey of life, single women often find themselves carrying emotional baggage from past traumas, childhood issues, heartbreaks, failed relationships, grief, loss, phobias, and fears. These burdens can weigh heavily on their hearts and hold them back from experiencing a fulfilling and joyful life. However, it is possible to heal and transform this baggage into something beautiful.

The first step towards ending meaning and moving forward is acknowledging and accepting the emotional baggage you carry. It is important to recognize that your past doesn't define you, but it has shaped you into the strong and resilient woman you are today. By acknowledging your experiences, you can begin the process of healing and letting go.

Healing from past trauma requires a combination of self-reflection, therapy, and self-care. It is essential to create a safe space to process your emotions, whether it be through journaling, counseling, or support groups. By facing your trauma head-on, you can begin to release the pain and find healing.

Coping with childhood issues may involve revisiting painful memories and understanding how they have influenced your present mindset and behaviors. Through therapy or self-help techniques, you can learn to reframe your past experiences and develop healthier coping mechanisms. Remember, you have the power to rewrite your story and create a brighter future.

Overcoming heartbreak and failed relationships can be emotionally challenging, but it is crucial to remember that these experiences do not determine your worth. Take the time to grieve, heal, and rediscover yourself. Focus on self-love and personal growth, and eventually, you will attract healthy and fulfilling relationships into your life.

Dealing with grief and loss requires patience and self-compassion. Allow yourself to mourn and honor your feelings. Seek support from loved ones or professional counselors who can guide you through the grieving process. Remember that healing takes time, and it is okay to take the necessary steps to move forward at your own pace.

Navigating through phobias and fears may seem daunting, but with determination and support, you can conquer them. Seek therapy or try techniques such as exposure therapy to gradually face your fears. Surround yourself with a supportive network that understands your journey and encourages your growth.

Finding meaning and moving forward is a journey unique to each individual. Embrace the process, be patient with yourself, and celebrate every small victory along the way. Remember that healing emotional baggage is not an overnight process, but with perseverance and self-compassion, you can transform your brokenness into something beautiful, ultimately leading to a life filled with joy, love, and purpose.

Chapter 6: Navigating Through Phobias and Fears

Exploring Common Phobias and Fears

Phobias and fears are common experiences that can greatly impact our lives, especially for single women who may be carrying emotional baggage from past traumas or dealing with childhood issues. In this subchapter, we will delve into the world of phobias and fears, understanding their origins and providing strategies for healing and overcoming them.

Phobias are irrational and intense fears that can cause significant distress and anxiety. They can range from common fears such as spiders or heights to more specific phobias like yin or public speaking. Many phobias stem from past traumas or childhood experiences, which have left deep emotional scars and triggered these irrational fears.

For single women carrying emotional baggage, exploring and understanding these phobias and fears is essential for healing and growth. By acknowledging and confronting them, we can begin the journey towards overcoming the limitations they impose on our lives.

In this subchapter, we will discuss various techniques and coping mechanisms to help single women navigate through their phobias and fears. We will explore therapeutic approaches such as cognitive-behavioral therapy (CBT), which helps individuals identify and challenge negative thought patterns associated with their fears. Additionally, we will delve into relaxation techniques, such as deep breathing exercises and mindfulness, to alleviate anxiety and promote a sense of calmness.

Furthermore, we will address the importance of seeking professional help when necessary. Sometimes, phobias and fears can be deeply rooted and require the guidance of a therapist or counselor to unravel their origins and develop effective strategies for healing.

By addressing and overcoming our phobias and fears, single women can regain control over their lives and break free from the limitations imposed by past traumas and childhood issues. This subchapter aims to empower women by providing them with the tools and knowledge necessary to navigate through their fears and emerge stronger and more resilient.

Whether it is overcoming heartbreak and failed relationships, dealing with grief and loss, or navigating through various phobias and fears, this subchapter seeks to support single women in their journey from brokenness to beauty. By healing emotional baggage, single women can embrace their true selves and create fulfilling lives, filled with love, joy, and personal growth.

Overcoming Phobias and Fears

Fear can be a paralyzing emotion that holds us back from living our lives to the fullest. Whether it's a phobia of spiders, heights, or public speaking, these fears can limit our potential and prevent us from experiencing new opportunities. In

In this subchapter, we will explore effective strategies to help single women overcome their phobias and fears, allowing them to break free from the chains of anxiety and embrace a life filled with courage and confidence.

Phobias and fears often stem from past traumas or childhood issues. It is crucial to understand the root cause of these fears in order to address them effectively. Through self-reflection and introspection, we can identify the triggering events or experiences that have contributed to the development of our phobias. By acknowledging and validating these emotions, we can begin the healing process and work towards overcoming them.

One effective approach to conquering phobias is through exposure therapy. Gradually exposing oneself to the feared object or situation in a controlled and supportive environment can help desensitize the fear response over time. Seeking professional guidance from therapists or joining support groups can provide the necessary tools and encouragement to face these fears head-on.

Another powerful tool in overcoming phobias is mindfulness and relaxation techniques. By practicing deep breathing exercises, meditation, and visualization, we can calm our anxious minds and reduce the intensity of our fears. Learning to reframe negative thoughts and replace them with positive affirmations can also help shift our mindset and empower us to confront our phobias with strength and resilience.

It is important to remember that overcoming phobias takes time and patience. Progress may be slow, but each small step forward is a victory worth celebrating. Surrounding oneself with a supportive network of friends, family, or fellow single women who understand the challenges of overcoming fears can provide invaluable encouragement and motivation along the journey.

As single women, we have already demonstrated immense strength and resilience in navigating through heartbreak, grief, and loss. Overcoming phobias and fears is yet another obstacle that we can conquer. By facing our fears head-on, we can reclaim our power and transform our lives from broken to beautiful. Let us embrace the journey of healing emotional baggage and emerge as courageous, confident, and fearless women who are ready to embrace all that life has to over.

From Broken to Beautiful: Healing Emotional Baggage for Single Women

From Broken to Beautiful: Healing Emotional Baggage for Single Women

Developing Resilience and Courage

In the journey from brokenness to beauty, developing resilience and courage is a crucial step for single women. Life throws various challenges our way, and it is our ability to bounce back and face them head-on that determines our emotional strength and overall well-being. This subchapter aims to provide guidance and practical strategies for single women to cultivate resilience and courage, enabling them to heal from emotional baggage and overcome past traumas.

Healing from past trauma often leaves emotional scars that can affect our relationships and overall happiness. By developing resilience, single women can learn to face these traumas and heal from them. It is important to acknowledge that healing takes time and effort, and it is a personal journey. By seeking professional help, joining support groups, or engaging in therapeutic activities such as journaling or art therapy, women can gradually heal and regain control over their lives.

Coping with childhood issues is another aspect that requires resilience and courage. Many single women carry unresolved childhood traumas that impact their self-esteem and relationships. It is vital to confront these issues and work through them. By seeking therapy or counseling, women can gain insight into their childhood experiences and learn healthy coping mechanisms that will enable them to navigate through life with strength and resilience.

Overcoming heartbreak and failed relationships is an inevitable part of life, but it does not define us. Developing resilience allows single women to bounce back from heartbreak, learning from past experiences and embracing the lessons they have learned. By focusing on self-care, self-love, and personal growth, women can build the courage to open their hearts again and create healthier and more fulfilling relationships.

Dealing with grief and loss is a universal experience, and it often tests our resilience. Single women may face the loss of loved ones, dreams, or opportunities. It is crucial to give oneself time and permission to grieve, while also finding healthy outlets for emotions such as engaging in support groups or seeking professional help. By developing resilience, women can honor their grief while also finding the strength to move forward and embrace new beginnings.

Navigating through phobias and fears can be challenging but not impossible. Resilience and courage empower single women to confront their fears, step out of their comfort zones, and grow. By seeking therapy or engaging in exposure therapy techniques, women can gradually overcome their phobias and fears, leading to a more fulfilling and fearless life.

In summary, developing resilience and courage is essential for single women to heal from emotional baggage, overcome past traumas, cope with childhood issues, navigate through heartbreak and failed relationships, deal with grief and loss, and conquer phobias and fears. By cultivating these qualities, women can transform their brokenness into beauty and create a life filled with strength, growth, and emotional well-being.

Chapter 7: Embracing Self-Love and Self-Care

Cultivating Self-Love and Acceptance

In the journey from brokenness to beauty, one of the most crucial steps for single women is cultivating self-love and acceptance. This subchapter aims to provide guidance and support for those dealing with emotional baggage, healing from past trauma, coping with childhood issues, overcoming heartbreak and failed relationships, dealing with grief and loss, and navigating through phobias and fears. By embracing self-love and acceptance, single women can create a solid foundation for their personal growth and journey towards healing.

Self-love is the foundation upon which all healing begins. It involves acknowledging and accepting oneself, aws and all. It is about recognizing one's worth and treating oneself with kindness, compassion, and respect. Through self-love, single women can start to release the emotional baggage that has burdened them for far too long.

Acceptance is an essential part of the healing process. It requires acknowledging the pain and trauma of the past without allowing it to define one's future. Acceptance allows single women to let go of the past and embrace the present moment. It is about learning to forgive oneself and others, releasing any resentment or anger that may be holding them back.

Healing from past trauma and coping with childhood issues can be a challenging process. However, by cultivating self-love and acceptance, single women can begin to unravel the layers of pain and find healing within themselves. It is important to seek professional help, if necessary, to guide them through this journey and provide tools to cope with the emotional challenges that may arise.

Heartbreak and failed relationships can leave deep scars, affecting one's self esteem and ability to trust again. By practicing self-love and acceptance, single women can rebuild their confidence and learn valuable lessons from past experiences. They can rediscover their worth and attract healthier, more fulfilling relationships in the future.

Dealing with grief and loss requires immense strength and self-compassion. By cultivating self-love and acceptance, single women can allow themselves to mourn and heal from the pain of loss. They can honor their emotions and give themselves permission to grieve, while also finding ways to cultivate self-care and self-nurturing practices.

Navigating through phobias and fears can be an overwhelming task. By embracing self-love and acceptance, single women can confront these fears with courage and compassion. They can seek support from therapists or support groups to develop coping mechanisms and strategies to overcome their fears.

In conclusion, cultivating self-love and acceptance is a vital step in the journey from brokenness to beauty for single women. By embracing these practices, they can release emotional baggage, heal from past trauma, cope with childhood issues, overcome heartbreak and failed relationships, deal with grief and loss, and navigate through phobias and fears. Through self-love and acceptance, single women can rebuild their lives, find inner strength, and create a future filled with love, joy, and fulfillment.

Practicing Self-Care Techniques

In the journey of healing emotional baggage, self-care is an essential tool for single women who aim to transform their brokenness into beauty. It is a powerful practice that helps them rejuvenate, restore, and nurture their emotional well-being. By engaging in self-care techniques, single women can address their emotional baggage, heal from past trauma, cope with childhood issues, overcome heartbreak and failed relationships, deal with grief and loss, as well as navigate through phobias and fears.

Self-care starts with acknowledging the importance of prioritizing oneself. As single women, it is easy to get caught up in the demands of work, relationships, and societal expectations. However, it is crucial to remember that taking care of one's own needs is not selfish, but rather a necessary step towards healing and growth. By setting aside dedicated time for self-care, single women can create a safe and nurturing space for themselves to heal and recharge.

There are numerous self-care techniques that can be incorporated into daily routines. Engaging in activities that bring joy, such as reading, painting, or dancing, can help single women reconnect with their inner selves and experience moments of tranquility. Physical exercise, whether through yoga, running, or any other form of movement, not only improves physical health but also releases endorphins, reducing stress and anxiety.

Practicing mindfulness and meditation is another powerful self-care technique that can help single women process their emotions and gain clarity. Taking time to react, journal, or engage in therapy can also provide a safe outlet for exploring and healing from past traumas, childhood issues, heartbreak, and failed relationships. Seeking support from trusted friends, family members, or professional therapists is essential in this process.

When dealing with grief and loss, self-care becomes even more crucial. Engaging in activities that honor and celebrate the memories of loved ones can help single women navigate through the grieving process. Similarly, when facing phobias and fears, self-care techniques such as exposure therapy, deep breathing exercises, and visualization can aid in overcoming these challenges.

By incorporating self-care techniques into their lives, single women can embark on a transformative journey from brokenness to beauty. They can heal their emotional baggage, overcome past traumas, cope with childhood issues, navigate heartbreak, deal with grief and loss, and conquer their phobias and fears. Through self-care, they can cultivate self-love, resilience, and a deep sense of empowerment. Ultimately, practicing self-care becomes an act of self love, paving the way for a beautiful and fulfilling life.

Building a Supportive Network

In the journey of healing emotional baggage, building a supportive network is an essential step for single women. This subchapter aims to guide you on how to establish a strong support system that will aid in your healing process and provide a safe space for growth and transformation. Whether you are dealing with past trauma, coping with childhood issues, overcoming heartbreak and failed relationships, dealing with grief and loss, or navigating through phobias and fears, a supportive network can be your lifeline.

Healing from emotional baggage can often feel like a daunting task, but with the right people by your side, you will find strength and comfort. Surrounding yourself with individuals who understand and empathize with your struggles can make a world of difference. Seek out friends, family members, or support

groups that specialize in emotional healing or share similar experiences. These individuals can over a listening ear, provide guidance, and share their own stories of triumph over adversity.

In addition to personal connections, consider seeking professional help. Therapists, counselors, or life coaches who specialize in healing from past trauma or overcoming emotional challenges can provide invaluable support. They can help you navigate through the complexities of your emotions, guide you towards healing, and equip you with coping strategies to overcome your specific issues.

It is also important to remember that building a supportive network goes beyond seeking help from others. It involves self-care and self-reflection. Take the time to identify your needs and set boundaries that protect your emotional well-being. Surround yourself with individuals who uplift and inspire you, rather than those who drain your energy.

Moreover, don't be afraid to reach out to others who have walked a similar path. Joining support groups or online communities can connect you with individuals who have overcome similar challenges. Sharing your experiences and hearing others' stories can foster a sense of belonging, reduce feelings of isolation, and inspire hope.

Building a supportive network is an ongoing process. As you heal and grow, your needs may change, and your network should adapt accordingly. Be open to new connections, and don't hesitate to lean on your support system during difficult times.

Remember, you are not alone in your journey. By building a supportive network, you are equipping yourself with the tools and resources necessary to transform from broken to beautiful. Embrace the power of connection and allow others to walk alongside you on the path to healing.

Chapter 8: Creating a Vision for the Future

Setting Goals and Intentions

In our journey from brokenness to beauty, setting goals and intentions becomes a crucial step towards healing emotional baggage for single women. Often, we carry the weight of past trauma, childhood issues, heartbreak, failed relationships, grief, loss, and even phobias and fears. However, by focusing on our goals and intentions, we can begin to navigate through these challenges and reclaim our strength and joy.

The first step is to acknowledge the emotional baggage we carry. It's important to recognize that it is not our fault and that we have the power to heal and move forward. By setting goals, we create a roadmap towards healing and transformation. These goals can be small or big, but they should be realistic and achievable. For instance, setting a goal to attend therapy or seeking support from a support group can be a significant step in healing from past trauma.

Intentions, on the other hand, are the guiding principles that help us stay focused on our goals. They are the values and beliefs that guide our actions. For example, if one of our goals is to overcome heartbreak and failed relationships, our intention could be to cultivate self-love and prioritize our own well-being. By setting this intention, we remind ourselves to take care of our emotional needs, to practice self-compassion, and to surround ourselves with positive influences.

When setting goals and intentions, it's crucial to be patient and kind to ourselves. Healing emotional baggage is a process, and it takes time. We may face setbacks and obstacles along the way, but by staying committed to our goals and intentions, we can overcome them. Celebrating small victories is also important to keep our motivation and momentum going.

Additionally, it can be helpful to seek support from others who have gone through similar experiences. Connecting with a community of single women who are also healing from emotional baggage can provide a sense of belonging, understanding, and encouragement. Sharing our stories and learning from each other's journeys can be empowering and inspiring.

In conclusion, setting goals and intentions is a powerful tool for single women who are healing from emotional baggage. It helps us navigate through past trauma, childhood issues, heartbreak, failed relationships, grief, loss, phobias, and fears. By setting realistic goals and aligning them with our guiding intentions, we can take charge of our healing journey and transform our brokenness into beauty. Remember, be patient, kind to yourself, and seek support from a community that understands your experiences. You are strong, resilient, and capable of reclaiming your joy and living a beautiful life.

Designing a Life of Purpose and Fulfillment

In the journey of life, many single women find themselves burdened with emotional baggage from past experiences. Whether it is trauma, childhood issues, heartbreak, failed relationships, grief, or phobias and fears, these emotional wounds can hinder personal growth and fulfillment. However, it is possible to break free from the chains of the past and design a life of purpose and fulfillment.

Healing from emotional baggage requires a deep understanding of oneself and a commitment to personal growth. It starts with acknowledging the pain and trauma that has been endured and facing it head-on. By seeking professional help or joining support groups, single women can find a safe space to express their emotions and begin the healing process.

Coping with childhood issues is an essential part of the journey towards a fulfilling life. Childhood experiences shape our beliefs and behaviors, often unconsciously. By uncovering and understanding these patterns, single women can break free from negative cycles and create healthier relationships and lifestyles.

Overcoming heartbreak and failed relationships is a significant challenge for many single women. It is crucial to realize that these experiences do not define one's worth or future. Learning to let go, forgiving oneself and others, and embracing the lessons learned can lead to personal growth and ultimately, finding a fulfilling and loving relationship.

Dealing with grief and loss is an inevitable part of life. Whether it is the loss of a loved one or dreams that did not come true, grief can be overwhelming. Single women need support and understanding during these times, allowing themselves to grieve and heal at their own pace. By using healthy coping mechanisms and seeking professional help if needed, it is possible to navigate through grief and find joy again.

Navigating through phobias and fears is another hurdle on the path to a fulfilling life. Identifying the root cause of these fears and challenging them gradually can lead to personal growth and expanded horizons. Facing fears head-on and seeking support from trusted individuals can empower single women to overcome limitations and live a life filled with purpose and fulfillment.

Designing a life of purpose and fulfillment is a personal journey that requires self-reflection, healing, and self-discovery. By addressing emotional baggage, healing from past trauma, coping with childhood issues, overcoming heartbreak and failed relationships, dealing with grief and loss, and navigating through phobias and fears, single women can create a life that is authentic, meaningful, and filled with joy. Remember, it is never too late to embark on this journey and design the life you deserve.

Embracing Growth and Transformation

Embracing growth and transformation is a crucial step in the journey of healing emotional baggage for single women. It is an empowering process that allows us to break free from the shackles of our past and step into a brighter, more fulfilling future.

Healing from past trauma is an essential aspect of this transformation. Many single women carry emotional baggage from past experiences that continue to impact their lives and relationships. By acknowledging and addressing these traumas, we can begin to release their hold on us and create space for healing and growth.

Coping with childhood issues can be particularly challenging, as the wounds from our formative years often shape our beliefs and behaviors as adults. However, by delving into these issues with compassion and understanding, we can gain valuable insights into ourselves and begin to rewrite the narratives that no longer serve us.

Overcoming heartbreak and failed relationships is another significant hurdle that single women often face. It is essential to recognize that these experiences do not define us but instead provide opportunities for growth and self discovery. By embracing the lessons learned from these relationships, we can become stronger and more resilient individuals.

Dealing with grief and loss is a universal experience, and as single women, we may find ourselves navigating through this process alone. It is crucial to allow ourselves to grieve fully and seek support when needed. Embracing growth and transformation means honoring our emotions and taking the necessary steps towards healing and finding new meaning in life.

Navigating through phobias and fears is also an essential part of this journey. Many single women may have developed fears and phobias as a result of their past experiences. By facing these fears head-on and seeking professional help if necessary, we can gradually overcome them and reclaim our power.

Embracing growth and transformation requires courage and perseverance. It is not always an easy path, but it is one that promises immense rewards. By actively engaging in self-reflection, seeking support, and embracing new opportunities, single women can heal their emotional baggage and create a beautiful, fulfilling life.

In the following chapters, we will explore various strategies, techniques, and stories of resilience from single women who have successfully embraced growth and transformation. Together, we will discover the transformative power of healing emotional baggage and embark on a journey towards personal growth, self-love, and the beautiful life we deserve.

Chapter 9: Maintaining Emotional Well-being

Implementing Stress Reduction Techniques

In today's fast-paced society, stress has become an unavoidable part of our lives. For single women who are already dealing with emotional baggage, past trauma, heartbreak, grief, and various fears, stress can feel overwhelming. However, it is crucial to prioritize our mental and emotional well-being and

find effective ways to manage stress. In this subchapter, we will explore some powerful stress reduction techniques that can help single women on their journey from broken to beautiful.

1. Mindfulness and Meditation: Practicing mindfulness and meditation can bring immense benefits to our mental and emotional health. By living in the present moment and focusing on our breath, we can calm our racing thoughts and find inner peace. Regular meditation can also improve our ability to cope with stress and cultivate a positive mindset.

2. Physical Exercise: Engaging in regular physical exercise is not only essential for our physical health but also for managing stress. Exercise releases endorphins, the feel-good hormones, which can uplift our mood and reduce anxiety. Whether it's going for a walk, practicing yoga, or hitting the gym,

finding an exercise routine that suits your preferences can be incredibly beneficial.

3. Deep Breathing: When stress strikes, taking a moment to practice deep breathing can work wonders. Deep breathing exercises activate the body's relaxation response, reducing stress hormones and promoting a sense of

calmness. By focusing on our breath and inhaling deeply through our nose and exhaling slowly through our mouth, we can instantly alleviate stress.

4. Self-Care Activities: Engaging in self-care activities is crucial for single women who are healing from past trauma and navigating through heartbreak and failed relationships. Taking time for oneself, whether it's indulging in a bubble bath, reading a book, practicing a hobby, or spending time in nature, can help to reduce stress levels and promote emotional well-being.

5. Seeking Support: Dealing with emotional baggage, childhood issues, grief, and fears can feel isolating, but remember, you are not alone. Seek support from trusted friends, family members, or even professional therapists or support groups. Sharing your emotions and experiences with others can provide a sense of relief and help you gain new perspectives on your journey to healing.

By implementing these stress reduction techniques into your daily routine, you can effectively manage stress, enhance your emotional well-being, and cultivate a life that is fulfilling and beautiful. Remember, healing is a process, and it takes time, but with dedication and self-care, you can overcome the challenges and emerge stronger on the other side.

Nurturing Emotional Health

Emotional health is a crucial aspect of our overall well-being, and for single women who may have experienced past trauma, heartbreak, or loss, it becomes even more important to prioritize self-care and healing. In this subchapter, we will explore various strategies and practices to nurture your emotional health and help you move from a place of brokenness to beauty.

Healing from past trauma can be a challenging journey, but it is essential for your emotional well-being. Acknowledging your pain and seeking professional help, such as therapy or support groups, can be a transformative step towards healing. By addressing the root causes of your trauma, you can start to regain control over your life and build a foundation for emotional resilience.

Coping with childhood issues is another area that many single women may need to address. Childhood experiences can have a profound impact on our emotional health, shaping our beliefs, behaviors, and relationships. Through self-reflection and therapy, you can begin to understand and heal from any

unresolved childhood wounds, paving the way for healthier relationships and a more fulfilling life.

Overcoming heartbreak and failed relationships is a common struggle for many single women. It is important to give yourself time and space to grieve and heal, while also cultivating self-love and self-compassion. Engaging in activities that bring you joy, surrounding yourself with a supportive community, and practicing self-care can aid in the healing process, allowing you to move forward with a renewed sense of hope.

Dealing with grief and loss is another emotional challenge that many single women face. Whether it is the loss of a loved one, a job, or a dream, the grieving process can be overwhelming. It is essential to honor your feelings and allow yourself to grieve in your own way. Seeking professional help or joining a grief support group can provide valuable guidance and comfort during this difficult time.

Navigating through phobias and fears is yet another aspect of nurturing your emotional health. Fear can hold us back from living our fullest lives, and it is important to confront and overcome these fears. Working with a therapist or

A coach who specializes in anxiety and fear can help you develop coping mechanisms and strategies to gradually face your fears, allowing you to expand your comfort zone and embrace new opportunities.

In conclusion, nurturing your emotional health is a vital step towards healing emotional baggage for single women. By addressing past trauma, coping with childhood issues, overcoming heartbreak and failed relationships, dealing with grief and loss, and navigating through phobias and fears, you can embark on a

journey of self-discovery, healing, and personal growth. Remember, you are capable of transforming your brokenness into something beautiful, and by prioritizing your emotional well-being, you can create a life of fulfillment, joy, and love.

Establishing Healthy Boundaries

In the journey of healing emotional baggage, one of the most crucial steps for single women is establishing healthy boundaries. Boundaries act as protective shields, safeguarding our emotional well-being and allowing us to navigate relationships with confidence and self-respect. They serve as a powerful tool for healing from past trauma, coping with childhood issues, overcoming heartbreak, dealing with grief and loss, and navigating through phobias and fears.

Setting boundaries can be challenging, especially if you have never prioritized your own needs or have had experiences that made you question your worth. However, it is an essential step towards reclaiming your power and creating a life filled with love, joy, and fulfillment.

To establish healthy boundaries, begin by understanding your own values, desires, and limits. Reflect on what feels comfortable and uncomfortable for you in various aspects of your life, such as relationships, work, and personal space. This self-awareness will serve as a foundation for asserting your boundaries confidently.

Next, communicate your boundaries clearly and assertively. Remember, your needs are valid, and it is essential to express them without guilt or fear of rejection. Practice saying "no" when something doesn't align with your values or makes you uncomfortable. It is not selfish to put yourself first; it is an act of self-care and self-respect.

Be prepared for resistance or pushback from others, especially those who have become accustomed to you not having boundaries. Stand firm and remember that you deserve to be treated with respect and kindness. Surround yourself with supportive individuals who honor and respect your boundaries.

Additionally, practice self-care regularly to reinforce your boundaries. Prioritize activities that nourish your mind, body, and soul. Engage in therapy or counseling to heal past wounds and gain tools to navigate through life's challenges. Seek out support groups or networks where you can connect with others who have similar experiences and learn from their journeys.

Lastly, be patient with yourself. Establishing healthy boundaries is a process that takes time and practice. There may be setbacks along the way, but each step you take towards honoring and protecting your emotional well-being is a step towards healing and finding true happiness.

Remember, as a single woman healing from emotional baggage, establishing healthy boundaries is a powerful act of self-love. It empowers you to create a life filled with authentic connections, emotional freedom, and personal growth. Embrace this journey and watch as you transform from broken to beautiful.

Chapter 10: Celebrating Your Journey

Reflecting on Personal Growth

In our journey through life, personal growth is an essential component that allows us to heal emotional baggage and transform ourselves from broken to beautiful. As single women, we often carry the weight of past traumas, childhood issues, heartbreak, failed relationships, grief, loss, phobias, and fears. However, it is through reflection and introspection that we can overcome these challenges and emerge stronger, wiser, and more resilient.

Reflecting on personal growth starts with acknowledging our emotional baggage. We must be willing to delve deep into our past, understanding the experiences that have shaped us and the wounds that still linger. It is not an easy task, but by facing our past head-on, we can begin the process of healing.

Healing from past trauma is a crucial step in our personal growth journey. It requires us to be gentle with ourselves, allowing time and space for the wounds to heal. Seeking therapy, support groups, or engaging in self-help practices can provide valuable tools to navigate this healing process. By addressing our trauma, we can gradually release its grip on our lives and create space for new beginnings.

Coping with childhood issues is another aspect that demands our attention. Childhood experiences often shape our relationships and how we perceive ourselves. Reflecting on these issues allows us to identify patterns and behaviors that may be holding us back. By understanding the root causes of our childhood issues, we can consciously break free from negative cycles and cultivate healthier relationships, both with ourselves and others.

Overcoming heartbreak and failed relationships is an inevitable part of life. It is during these moments of profound pain that personal growth truly shines. Reflecting on these experiences allows us to learn valuable lessons about love, resilience, and self-worth. By embracing our vulnerability, we can rebuild our lives and open ourselves to the possibility of new, healthier relationships.

Dealing with grief and loss is a deeply personal journey that requires time and compassion. Reflecting on our grief allows us to honor our emotions and find ways to heal. Connecting with support networks, seeking therapy, or engaging in creative outlets can provide solace and help us navigate the grieving process.

Navigating through phobias and fears is an integral part of personal growth. Reflecting on the origins of these fears allows us to confront them head-on and challenge their hold over us. With courage and determination, we can gradually overcome these obstacles, expand our comfort zones, and embrace a life filled with freedom and fulfillment.

In conclusion, reflecting on personal growth is a transformative process that empowers single women to heal emotional baggage, overcome past traumas, cope with childhood issues, navigate heartbreak and failed relationships, deal

with grief and loss, and conquer phobias and fears. By embarking on this journey of self-discovery, we can emerge from brokenness to embrace our inner beauty, strength, and resilience.

Embracing the Beauty of Healing

Healing is a transformative and empowering journey that holds the key to unlocking your true potential. As single women, we often carry emotional baggage from past experiences that can hinder our growth and prevent us from fully embracing life's beautiful opportunities. In this subchapter, "Embracing the Beauty of Healing," we will explore the various facets of healing emotional baggage, and how it can help us overcome the challenges we face.

One of the first steps in healing is acknowledging and understanding our emotional baggage. We all carry wounds from past trauma, childhood issues, heartbreaks, failed relationships, grief, loss, phobias, and fears. These experiences shape our perceptions of ourselves and the world around us. By delving deep into these emotional wounds, we can begin to untangle the roots of our pain and start the healing process.

Healing from past trauma is a complex and individual journey. It requires a combination of self-reflection, therapy, and support from loved ones. By addressing the trauma head-on, we can release the negative energy associated with it and create space for healing and personal growth. It is through this healing that we can break free from the chains of our past and create a brighter future.

Coping with childhood issues is another crucial aspect of healing emotional baggage. Our childhood experiences shape our beliefs, self-worth, and ability to form healthy relationships. By recognizing the impact of these issues, we can work towards healing the wounds that still affect us today. Through therapy, self-care, and self-compassion, we can learn to reframe our mindset and develop healthier coping mechanisms.

Heartbreaks and failed relationships can leave us feeling shattered and doubtful about love. However, healing from these experiences is possible. By embracing the pain, allowing ourselves to grieve, and learning from our past relationships, we can grow stronger and wiser. Healing allows us to let go of bitterness and open ourselves up to new possibilities and healthier relationships in the future.

Dealing with grief and loss is an inevitable part of life. The healing process requires us to honor our emotions, seek support, and find healthy ways to remember and cherish our loved ones. Healing does not mean forgetting; it means finding peace and acceptance within ourselves, even in the face of loss.

Navigating through phobias and fears can be a daunting task, but healing can help us face these challenges head-on. By recognizing the root causes of our fears and seeking therapy or professional help, we can gradually overcome them. Healing allows us to reclaim our power and live a life free from the limitations that fear imposes.

Embracing the beauty of healing is a transformative journey that single women can embark on to release emotional baggage and forge a path towards a more fulfilling life. By acknowledging our past, seeking support, and embracing self care, we can heal, grow, and blossom into our most beautiful selves. The journey may be challenging, but the rewards are immeasurable. Remember, healing is not a destination; it is a lifelong commitment to ourselves and our well-being.

Inspiring and Supporting Others

In our journey towards healing emotional baggage, it is essential to remember that our experiences are not isolated. As single women, we have the power to inspire and support others who may be going through similar struggles. By sharing our stories and offering guidance, we can create a community of strength and resilience.

Healing from past trauma can be a daunting task, but it becomes more manageable when we come together in solidarity. As we navigate through our own emotional baggage, we can extend a helping hand to those who may be struggling with their own past traumas. By sharing our healing strategies and offering a listening ear, we can provide a safe space for others to open up and begin their journey towards wholeness.

Coping with childhood issues is another area where our support can make a significant impact. Many of us carry wounds from our formative years that continue to affect our present lives. By sharing our coping mechanisms and offering guidance, we can empower other single women to confront their childhood issues head-on. Together, we can break free from the chains of the past and create a brighter future.

Heartbreak and failed relationships can leave us feeling shattered and defeated. However, as single women who have experienced these painful emotions, we have the power to inspire others to rise above their heartbreak. By sharing our stories of resilience and showcasing the strength we discovered within ourselves, we can motivate others to continue their journey towards self-love and personal growth.

Dealing with grief and loss is an integral part of the healing process. As single women, we have the ability to support others who may be grieving the loss of a loved one or experiencing the pain of a broken dream. By offering a shoulder to lean on and sharing our own experiences of navigating through grief, we can provide solace and encouragement to those who need it most.

Navigating through phobias and fears is yet another aspect of healing that we can address as single women. Many of us battle with deep-rooted fears that hinder our personal growth and happiness. By sharing our strategies for conquering phobias and fears, we can inspire others to face their own anxieties head-on. Together, we can create a supportive network where no fear is insurmountable.

In conclusion, as single women healing from emotional baggage, we have the power to inspire and support others in their own journey towards wholeness. By sharing our stories, offering guidance, and creating a community of strength, we can empower each other to overcome past traumas, cope with childhood issues, heal from heartbreak and failed relationships, deal with grief and loss, and navigate through phobias and fears. Together, we can transform our brokenness into beauty and emerge as stronger, more resilient individuals.

Conclusion: Embracing Your Beautiful, Healed Self

As we reach the conclusion of this transformative journey, it is essential to react to the progress we have made as single women in healing our emotional baggage. From broken to beautiful, we have peeled back layers of pain, trauma, and heartbreak to uncover the resilient, courageous, and beautiful souls that reside within us.

Throughout this book, we have delved into various aspects of healing, addressing emotional baggage, and navigating through life's challenges. We have explored the depths of our past traumas, coping with childhood issues, overcoming heartbreak and failed relationships, dealing with grief and loss, and navigating through phobias and fears. Each step of this journey has been crucial in our growth and transformation.

It is important to acknowledge that healing is a continuous process. We must embrace the fact that our past may have shaped us, but it does not define us. We have the power to break free from the chains of our past and create a future filled with love, joy, and fulfillment.

As single women, we often carry a heavy burden of societal expectations and norms. We may feel pressured to conform, find a partner, or define our worth through external validation. However, true healing lies in embracing our unique journeys and loving ourselves unconditionally.

By healing our emotional baggage, we have gained a profound understanding of our own strengths and weaknesses. We have learned to set boundaries, prioritize self-care, and surround ourselves with positive influences. Through these practices, we create a solid foundation for our future relationships, ensuring that they are built on love, respect, and mutual growth.

As we close this chapter, let us remember that healing is a lifelong commitment. It requires patience, self-compassion, and a willingness to confront our deepest fears and insecurities. By doing so, we open ourselves up to a world of endless possibilities, where we can thrive as beautiful, healed individuals.

May this book serve as a guide and a source of inspiration for all single women who are ready to embark on their healing journey. Embrace your beautiful, healed self, and remember that you are worthy of love, happiness, and fulfillment. Trust in your strength, believe in your resilience, and know that you have the power to transform your life from broken to truly beautiful.

From Broken to Beautiful: Healing Emotional Baggage for Single Women

Proverbs 31:10-31

A wife of noble character who can be found? She is worth far more than rubies. 11 Her husband has full confidence in her and lacks nothing of value. 12 She brings him good, not harm, all the days of her life. 13 She selects wool and

ax and works with eager hands. 14 She is like the merchant ships, bringing her food from afar. 15 She gets up while it is still night; she provides food for her family and portions for her female servants. 16 She considers a field and buys it; out of her earnings she plants a vineyard. 17 She sets about her work vigorously; her arms are strong for her tasks. 18 She sees that her trading is profitable, and her lamp does not go out at night. 19 In her hand she holds the distaff and grasps the spindle with her fingers. 20 She opens her arms to the poor and extends her hands to the needy. 21 When it snows, she has no fear for her household; for all of them are clothed in scarlet. 22 She makes coverings for her bed; she is clothed in fine linen and purple. 23 Her